T0144678

BASIC HEALTH
PUBLICATIONS
USER'S GUIDE

TO POLICOSANOL & OTHER NATURAL WAYS TO LOWER CHOLESTEROL

Learn about the Many Safe Ways to Reduce Your Cholesterol and Lower Your Risk of Heart Disease.

MARK STENGLER, N.D.

JACK CHALLEM Series Editor

The information contained in this book is based upon the research and personal and professional experiences of the author. It is not intended as a substitute for consulting with your physician or other healthcare provider. Any attempt to diagnose and treat an illness should be done under the direction of a healthcare professional.

The publisher does not advocate the use of any particular healthcare protocol but believes the information in this book should be available to the public. The publisher and author are not responsible for any adverse effects or consequences resulting from the use of the suggestions, preparations, or procedures discussed in this book. Should the reader have any questions concerning the appropriateness of any procedures or preparations mentioned, the author and the publisher strongly suggest consulting a professional healthcare advisor.

Series Editor: Jack Challem
Editor: Stephany Evans
Typesetter: Gary A. Rosenberg
Series Cover Designer: Mike Stromberg

Basic Health Publications, Inc.

ISBN: 978-1-59120-051-2 (Pbk.)
ISBN: 978-1-68162-866-0 (Hardcover)

CONTENTS

INTRODUCTION

Heart disease. We all know someone who either lives with it or who has died from it. Perhaps you have been told that you have heart disease, often referred to as cardiovascular disease (a term that recognizes the involvement of the entire heart and circulatory system).

More than 960,000 Americans succumb to cardiovascular disease each year. This staggering statistic accounts for approximately 41 percent of all deaths in the United States.

While cholesterol-lowering drugs and surgery are the favored therapy by conventional doctors, these alone are no longer considered the best medicine.

Tens of thousands of American health professionals are increasingly recommending dietary and lifestyle changes, which have been proven to make a dramatic impact on one's cardiovascular health, as well as nutritional supplements to prevent and reverse heart disease.

Does this natural approach work? You bet. And the risk of side effects is virtually nonexistent when compared with pharmaceutical and surgical options.

High cholesterol levels have long been vilified as the cause of most cases of heart disease. It's true that elevated levels can increase a person's risk of heart disease. Yet the potential toxicity of many cholesterol-lowering drugs have encouraged many to seek a better way to "normalize" cholesterol levels.

Specific nutritional supplements have been discovered that can work as well as highly publicized cholesterol drugs. Although your doctor may not recommend these natural cholesterol-lowering nutrients, many have substantial scientific studies to back up their effectiveness and safety.

One such natural supplement that effectively normalizes cholesterol levels and other markers for heart disease is Policosanol. And it works without the potentially fatal side effects you see with some cholesterol medications.

Because so much has been made of the issue, it may be surprising to learn that elevated cholesterol levels are only one small piece of the puzzle of why people develop heart disease. For example, in medical circles, it is a well-known fact that 50 percent of those who have heart attacks have *normal* cholesterol levels!

The *User's Guide to Policosanol and Other Natural Ways to Lower Cholesterol* was written to help people understand and effectively combat the causes of heart disease.

In Chapter 1, you will learn the mechanisms of how heart disease develops. I will also discuss the many risk factors associated with cardiovascular disease and what we can do to prevent them.

Chapter 2 focuses on the breakthrough supplement Policosanol. You will learn about the many ways it helps prevent and reverse heart disease. Included in Chapter 3 are numerous human studies that demonstrate its mechanism of action, effectiveness and safety, and how to use it.

Chapter 4 addresses the importance of dietary and lifestyle approaches in preventing and revers-ing heart disease.

The final chapters provide important recommendations on a variety of heart-healthy supplements to meet your individual health needs.

I hope you will be as enthusiastic as I am about the information in this book: it can improve the quality and length of your life. Enjoy.

CHAPTER 1

UNDERSTANDING HEART DISEASE

The heart, without a doubt, is one of the most incredible organs in the human body. This fist-sized organ pumps enough blood through the blood vessels to nourish and sustain all the trillions of cells in your body. Some experts believe that, under ideal circumstances, the heart can maintain its incredible pace for up to 120 years!

Providing proper nutrients is the key to a healthy heart and circulatory system, enabling them to work efficiently. In addition, one should avoid harmful lifestyle choices such as eating unhealthy fast food and smoking, which put undue stress on the heart.

However, there are also independent genetic risk factors that research has shown to greatly increase the odds of a cardiovascular disease. These genetic factors can be fatal even if one is following a healthy diet and lifestyle.

What Is Heart Disease?

"Heart disease" simply refers to a disorder of the heart. Many people use this as a general term to refer to the entire heart and circulatory system. A better term to cover the entire system of the heart and blood vessels is "cardiovascular disease."

Concomitant with cardiovascular disease is what is commonly called "hardening of the arteries," that is, arteriosclerosis. In this condition,

artery walls thicken and lose their flexibility, inter-
fering with circulation. The most common type of
arteriosclerosis is known as atherosclerosis. This
is an accumulation of fatty deposits along blood
vessel walls, resulting in a thickening and hardening of the medium to large artery walls.

Forms of Cardiovascular Disease

Many different conditions fall under the category
of cardiovascular disease. These conditions are
discussed below.

Myocardial Infarction

This is the medical term for a heart attack. This
occurs when too little oxygenated blood reaches
the heart, resulting in the death of heart tissue.
Arteries that have become clogged with fatty
deposits or a blood clot that has lodged in the
heart may cause a heart attack.

Characteristic symptoms include a squeezing
or sharp pain in the chest or upper abdomen.
The pain may radiate down the left or right arm
and into the neck, back, or shoulders. Shortness
of breath, faintness, nausea, and excessive per-
spiration are also common symptoms. It's possible to have a heart attack and mistake it for
indigestion, as the symptoms can be very similar.

Hypertension

One of the biggest risk factors for heart disease
is hypertension, also known as high blood pressure. This refers to the pressure inside the artery
walls. A normal reading is 120/80 mm/Hg. Sys-
tolic blood pressure (the first number) that is 140
and higher, and diastolic readings (the second
number) of 90 or more are considered to be elevated. If on three separate occasions you have an
elevated reading, your doctor will confirm a diagnosis of hypertension.

Stroke

This refers to brain damage caused by a lack of blood flow to a part of the brain. When blood flow is cut off to the brain, it prevents oxygen and nutrients from getting to brain tissue, which can lead to the death of brain cells.

Stroke is the third leading cause of death and a leading cause of serious, long-term disability in the United States. According to the American Heart Association, about 600,000 Americans suffer a stroke each year. Approximately 25 percent of these strokes are fatal.

Arrhythmia

Abnormal rhythm of the heart is known as an arrhythmia. There are many different types of arrhythmias with varying degrees of severity.

Symptoms may include heart palpitations, dizziness, or fainting. In more extreme cases, arrhythmia can result in death.

Valvular Disease

Valves of the heart help control blood flow. When they do not open or close properly, it can negatively affect blood flow. The severity of valve disease can widely vary.

Shortness of breath, heart palpitations, and chest pain can be symptoms of valvular disease. Most cases are not life threatening.

Murmur

Not actually a disease in itself, a "murmur" refers to the sound a doctor can hear when heart valves do not shut properly or when there is restricted blood flow through the heart. The seriousness of murmurs varies greatly.

Congestive Heart Failure

When the heart begins to fail as a pump, it is known as congestive heart failure. Years of high blood pressure or arteriosclerosis can lead to an inefficient pumping action of the heart. Symptoms may include fatigue, shortness of breath, and fluid retention in the lungs and legs.

What Causes Cardiovascular Disease?

Cardiovascular disease is not a condition that develops over the course of a few days or months. Generally speaking, it is the result of years of inflammation and damage to the blood vessel walls. This results in plaque formation and eventual blockage of blood flow through the arteries, and throughout the cardiovascular system, including the coronary arteries that supply oxygen and nutrients to the heart tissue. In this condition, one is more susceptible to a heart attack or stroke.

There are many different causes of plaque formation in the arteries. In recent years, it has become evident that chronic inflammation of the blood vessel walls is a common underlying theme in the development of heart disease. This inflammation accelerates the formation of plaque buildup in the arteries. The obvious question is, "What initiates the inflammation in one's arteries in the first place?"

Risk Factors for Heart Disease

To answer this question, we must examine the many risk factors for heart disease. These risk factors include diet and lifestyle choices. They also include genetic risk markers that your doctor can test you for. The good news is that all of these factors can be modified through dietary, lifestyle, and nutritional supplement choices.

Diet

One of the most powerful ways you can prevent and treat heart disease is through the foods you eat. Everyday choices we make for meals and snacks can make the difference as to whether our heart is healthy or diseased ten to twenty years from now.

I would hope that the days of the low-fat, high-carbohydrate diet to prevent and treat heart disease are over. This approach, which has been recommended by cardiologists over the past decade, is fast losing credibility. In fact, for some people, this approach actually increases their body weight, elevates cholesterol and other heart disease risk markers, and accelerates the progression of blocked arteries.

In Chapter 4, I will go into more detail about what types of foods you should be eating to prevent heart disease. For now, I will say only that research has shown that through proper diet one can reverse plaque buildup in the arteries. So, if you already have been diagnosed with arteriosclerosis, or hardening of the arteries, it is not too late.

Age

As with most health conditions, statistics demonstrate that the risk of heart disease increases with age. Approximately 80 percent of people who die of heart disease are age sixty-five and older.

The good news is that cardiovascular disease is not inevitable as you age. By addressing all the factors involved with heart disease, you can minimize the effects of aging on the heart.

Gender

Statistics show us that men have a greater risk of heart attack than do women. They also have heart attacks earlier in life. There are likely several reasons for this. For example, men tend to avoid going to the doctor for preventative exams. They also are more likely to internalize stress in their lives, which can contribute to negative changes in blood flow to the heart.

Heredity (Including Race)

If your parents had heart disease, you are more likely to develop it as well. Also, Black Americans tend to have more severe high blood pressure, which increases the risk of heart disease.

However, these factors do not make heart disease inevitable. Again, lifestyle modification can overcome these genetic susceptibilities. Part of the heredity factor is not genetic; families tend to follow the same diet and lifestyle traits throughout life, some of which can set one up for heart disease—like a junk food diet, for instance. Lifestyle choices such as smoking and overconsumption of alcohol also are big risk factors. In addition, poor stress coping skills can be passed on to children, which can increase their risk for disease. Thus, genetics are not really the culprit in many cases when there is a family history of heart disease.

Yet certain genetic markers are not greatly affected by diet and lifestyle and can be significant factors. These are discussed later in this chapter.

Stress

A high-stress lifestyle is an independent risk factor for heart disease. This includes sudden high-stress events, which may trigger a heart attack. Also, prolonged levels of stress cause elevation of the hormone cortisol. Elevated levels of this hormone over time leads to a breakdown of the immune and cardiovascular systems.

Depression has been shown to be a risk factor for heart disease. How one perceives and copes with stress is important as everyone is under a certain amount of stress. One study at the University of Maryland School of Medicine found that laughter and a good sense of humor provided significant protection against heart disease.

Stress coping mechanisms such as exercise,

deep breathing, prayer, time with family and friends, and many other methods work to reduce the disease-causing effects of stress.

Blood Markers: Predictors of Heart Disease

There are many blood markers that are used as predictors of heart disease. As you can see, cholesterol is only one small piece of the picture.

Cholesterol

This yellow, waxy substance is necessary for life. It is commonly portrayed as a villain to the heart. The reality, however, is that cholesterol is necessary for life. It is an essential component of every cell in your body.

Although cholesterol is present in some of the foods we eat, approximately 85 percent of cholesterol in your body is manufactured by your liver, and to a lesser degree, your small intestine.

The Framingham Study found that people with levels below 175 mg/dl had less than half the rate of heart attacks as those whose levels were 250–275 mg/dl.

Research over the past decade is showing that cholesterol's becoming oxidized is the real problem. Oxidation occurs when a person's antioxidant system cannot neutralize unstable, negatively charged molecules called free radicals. Oxidized cholesterol (particularly LDL cholesterol) then initiates inflammation of blood vessel walls, and an eventual buildup of plaque, which inhibits blood flow through the arteries.

Free Radicals
Unstable, negatively charged molecules that are potentially damaging to the organs and tissues of the body.

Interestingly, newer studies are showing that cholesterol-lowering statin drugs may have therapeutic benefits more because of their ability to reduce inflammation than because of their ability to lower cholesterol. Of course, inflammation can be reduced effectively with natural methods that do not come with the toxicity that sometimes occurs with these drugs.

High cholesterol levels can be, in some cases, a response to the inflammation of the cardiovascular system. However, there are many people who have very high levels of cholesterol due to genetics.

Total Cholesterol

The most nonspecific cholesterol marker is total cholesterol. While it is a risk marker worth following, studies are continuing to show it is less of a significant factor than once was previously thought. A healthy range is 175–200 mg/dL.

LDL (Low-Density Lipoprotein) Cholesterol

This cholesterol carries cholesterol from the liver to the blood vessel walls and cells of the body. It is often referred to as "bad cholesterol" because when LDL cholesterol becomes oxidized and attaches to the artery wall, it sets up a cascade of events that contributes to inflammation and plaque deposition. A healthy range is below 130 mg/dL.

HDL (High-Density Lipoprotein) Cholesterol

Often referred to by doctors as the "good cholesterol," HDL works to transport cholesterol from the artery walls to the liver to be metabolized. Elevated levels of HDL are desirable to offset the risks of elevated LDL. A healthy range is 50 mg/dL or higher.

Triglycerides

Fats in the blood, triglycerides either come from the diet or are manufactured by the liver. Eleva -

tions are common in those with increased blood sugar levels as seen in diabetes or insulin resistance. A high level of these fats can restrict blood flow and make one more susceptible to stroke. A healthy range is less than 150 mg/dL.

Lipoprotein (a)

Also referred to as Lp(a), this is actually a more specific cholesterol marker and a stronger risk factor than LDL cholesterol. It is a strong genetic marker and an accurate predictor of heart disease. Abnormally high levels increase the likelihood of blood clots and plaque buildup in the arteries. Some studies show that cholesterol medications such as Mevacor and Zocor may actually increase Lp(a) levels. A healthy range is less than 32 mg/dL.

Homocysteine

This independent marker of heart disease has an interesting history. In 1969, Dr. Kilmer McCully of Harvard University proposed that levels of high homocysteine in the blood mainly caused cardiovascular disease. His idea was so revolutionary that he was asked to leave Harvard for this "radical" new theory. In the past decade, numerous studies have confirmed the damage of elevated homocysteine levels—exactly what Dr. McCully told the medical community three decades ago! Research shows that elevated homocysteine levels can increase the risk of stroke by 42 percent. It is also associated with diseases such as rheum - atoid arthritis and Alzheimer's disease.

Studies have confirmed elevated homocysteine levels to be a more important risk marker for heart disease than cholesterol. Buildup of this toxic metabolite occurs when the amino acid methionine is not properly metabolized. Approx - imately 5 to 10 percent of the population have elevated homocysteine levels due to genetics. For others, elevated levels can be related to B vitamin deficiencies or low thyroid function. A healthy range is less than 10 micro mol/L.

C-Reactive Protein

The new "smoking gun" when it comes to measurable heart disease blood markers is C-reactive protein. This is a measurement of inflammation in the body as well as the blood vessels. Many experts consider it to be the most significant predictive marker of heart disease. Elevations of this value can increase a person's risk of cardiovascular disease from two to five times that of someone who has a normal level. The Women's Health Study found it to be the best predictor of heart disease in women.

C-Reactive Protein
A marker of inflammation in the body.

This protein can disrupt fatty plaque buildup inside blood vessels, which can trigger a stroke or heart attack. It also increases the rate of LDL oxidation. Chronic infections can elevate levels of C-reactive protein. A healthy range is less than 1.69 mg/L.

Fibrinogen

It is important for our blood to clot so that we do not bleed to death from injuries or cuts. However, blood that clots too easily can be a problem as well. Fibrinogen plays an important role in blood clotting. Higher levels of this substance are more common in people who smoke, are overweight, have lipid imbalances, and/or have diabetes. Elevated levels of fibrinogen put one at significant risk of stroke and coronary artery disease. A healthy range is between 180 and 300 mg/dL.

Iron

Iron is one of those paradoxical nutrients. Too

little of it in the body and one can be become anemic and tired. Conversely, too much iron increases the production of free radicals and oxidative damage. For example, people with hemochromatosis, a genetic condition characterized by abnormally high iron levels, die at a much younger age of heart disease if not diagnosed.

Blood tests that measure iron, iron saturation, and ferritin can help your doctor screen you for iron overload. A healthy range is less than 150 mg/dL.

Ferritin
Iron storage levels in the body.

Glucose

Elevated blood sugar (glucose) levels predispose one to heart disease. This is commonly seen in people with diabetes who tend to die at an earlier age, especially if they have had poor blood sugar control in the past.

Insulin resistance is often involved in elevated blood sugar levels and is considered a prelude to diabetes. Elevated glucose levels often trigger a simultaneous increase in triglycerides. A healthy range is between 80 and 100 mg/dL.

Insulin

Insulin is a hormone, produced by the pancreas, that functions to transport blood sugar into the cells. In some people, due to genetic abnormalities, poor dietary choices, and nutritional deficiencies, cells become resistant to the

Insulin
A hormone produced by the pancreas, responsible for blood sugar regulation.

"transporting effects" of insulin, that is, the cells will resist accepting the insulin.

Insulin resistance is an increasingly accepted risk factor for heart disease. When production of this hormone spikes due to elevated blood sugar levels, the oxidation of cholesterol and inflammation in the blood vessels increases. A healthy range for insulin is between 4 and 15 micro mol (fasting).

Other Risk Factors

Besides what can be measured by blood tests that identify specific markers, the following five risk factors are every bit as important:

Nutritional Deficiencies

A number of nutritional deficiencies can make one more susceptible to cardiovascular disease. Insufficient amounts of antioxidants—vitamin C, vitamin E, selenium, carotenoids, coenzyme Q_{10} and many others (discussed in Chapter 4) that are very important in the prevention of cholesterol oxidation—can increase your risk for disease. B vitamins are also critical—they help to prevent the buildup of homocysteine. A nutrition-oriented doctor can measure the levels of these nutrients with blood or urine tests.

High Blood Pressure

Elevated blood pressure is a significant risk for cardiovascular disease. High pressure inside the

---

The Thyroid Connection

High cholesterol and homocysteine levels can be the result of low thyroid function. Studies show that even mildly low thyroid hormone levels can increase elevations in cholesterol. For example, in one study, people who had no thyroid gland and required hormone replacement were asked to stop taking their thyroid medicine. This resulted in a 100 percent increase in cholesterol and a 27 percent increase in homocysteine. After restarting the thyroid hormone medicine, levels of these two markers went back to normal within four to six weeks.

artery wall leads to damage and the deposition of plaque. This high pressure also damages the heart, making one more prone to heart attack and congestive heart failure. A healthy range is 100–120/60–80 mm/Hg.

Overweight

Being overweight increases the likelihood of insulin resistance, high blood pressure, and elevated triglycerides and cholesterol. The heart has to work a lot harder to pump blood to all the cells of the body. A healthy range is within 5 percent of ideal bodyweight.

Smoking

It has been said—and may even be true—that smoking has killed more people than all those killed in wars throughout world history.

Smoking increases the risk of coronary artery disease by three to six times that of nonsmokers. It also increases cardiovascular risk markers such as cholesterol oxidation, elevated C-reactive protein, and fibrinogen levels. Smoking also increases the burden of toxic metals in the body such as cadmium and arsenic, which damage the cardiovascular system. And it contributes to elevated blood pressure.

Keep in mind that when you are exposed to secondhand smoke you are at risk for the same damaging effects found in smokers.

Low Grade Infections

One of the newest theories as to why heart disease develops is a stealth infection in the body. Small bacteria and yeast overgrowth may cause inflammation in blood vessels, which

Stealth Infection
A hidden infection within the body.

sets up an inflammatory response. Research is preliminary but continued studies may show a significant connection.

CHAPTER 2

THE POLICOSANOL ANSWER

Policosanol (pronounced *polly-KOH-san-all*) is a nutritional supplement that is gaining the attention of doctors and natural healthcare enthusiasts around the world. This increasingly popular supplement can normalize cholesterol levels in a manner similar to the pharmaceutical cholesterol medications. Policosanol also reduces many other risk factors associated with heart disease. Incredibly, it offers these impressive benefits without side effects.

Policosanol has been shown to effectively reduce harmful LDL cholesterol by 25 to 30 percent and increase the good HDL cholesterol by 15 to 25 percent. Even better, it prevents LDL cholesterol from becoming oxidized, decreases lipoprotein (a), reduces blood clot formation, promotes circulation, and reduces inflammation in the artery walls.

What Exactly Is Policosanol?

Policosanol is a naturally occurring compound extracted from sugar-cane wax, beeswax, or rice-bran wax. Nearly all studies on Policosanol have used the sugar cane wax extract form. It was first discovered and researched in Cuba as an effective, natural substance to reduce elevated cholesterol levels.

Policosanol is a combination of long-chain fatty alcohol groups. One of the main fatty alcohols is octacosanol. Octacosanol has been used for many decades as a safe supplement to improve endurance and energy production. It is found in the rind and leaves of citrus fruits.

Policosanol contains several other long-chain fatty alcohols. The prefix "poli" signifies these multiple, related fatty alcohols that work together for a synergistic effect in the body to optimize cardiovascular health.

Good Fatty Alcohols?

Understandably, the term "fatty alcohol" may not elicit any visions of health. This is simply a biochemical term signifying that a compound has an alcohol (OH group) attached to the end of its carbon chain.

Actually, fatty alcohols are used in the body to manufacture the insulation around nerves (known as myelin), as well as other important substances in the body. These same fatty alcohols are converted into essential fatty acids that have numerous documented health benefits.

The Cuban Connection

Cuba's socialized medical system has quite a positive attribute: it embraces the research and use of natural substances. There are three main reasons for this. First, herbs and natural medicines are a part of the Cuban culture and heritage. Second, the Cuban government encourages the use of local medicinal substances because they are considerably less expensive than pharmaceutical medications. And third, any side effects of these natural substances are generally fewer and less serious than those of prescription drugs.

Policosanol has been the focus of research by Cuban doctors and scientists for decades, and has become a mainstay in the prevention and treatment of heart disease. Studies looking at more than 80,000 Cubans have demonstrated its effectiveness and safety in promoting cardio-vascular health. The Cuban success has spurred research worldwide on Policosanol. Currently, millions around the world are using Policosanol as a nonpharmaceutical way to normalize choles-terol levels and other cardiovascular risk markers.

Mechanism of Action

Policosanol has a different mechanism of action than commonly prescribed cholesterol-lowering "statin" drugs such as Mevacor, Pravachol, and Zocor. These "statin" drugs work by inhibiting the liver enzyme HMG CoA reductase. This is the en-zyme that helps the liver synthesize cholesterol.

Unfortunately, this can come at a price. Liver toxicity tops the list as the biggest concern with these medications. Also, this is the same enzyme that is involved in the synthesis of CoQ_{10}, a nutri-ent the heart and all the cells of the body use for energy production.

Policosanol also works to block the synthesis of cholesterol, but in a different way than statin drugs. It appears to have an indirect effect on cholesterol synthesis by decreasing liver production of cholesterol or by enhancing the liver's metabo-lism and breakdown of choles-terol. Policosanol also has been shown to promote the degra-dation of LDL cholesterol.

> **LDL Cholesterol**
> Low-density lipoprotein that transports cholesterol, proteins, fats, and fat-soluble vitamins to body cells.

Research is still continuing in an effort to dis-cover the exact mechanism by which Policosanol favorably modulates cholesterol levels.

More Than Cholesterol Reduction

One of the positive effects that excites me about Policosanol (besides its effectiveness on imbalanced cholesterol levels, and its impressive safety record) is its benefit against other factors that cause heart disease, which are discussed below.

Reduces Blood Clot Formation

In a recent study, Policosanol was shown to significantly reduce platelet aggregation. Platelets are the sticky cells that form blood clots. By preventing excessive clumping of these cells, Policosanol may reduce the formation of a serious blood clot.

The blood-thinning effect of Policosanol may be compared to that of aspirin. It has been shown that after two weeks of use, it significantly reduces the levels of thromboxanes in humans. Thromboxane is a chemical in the body that causes blood vessel constriction and clotting, which can lead to a stroke or heart attack.

Platelet Aggregation
The tendency of blood platelets to stick together, promoting blood clot formation.

Promotes Arterial Health

The thickening of artery walls restricts optimal blood flow. This arterial wall thickening occurs when cells proliferate too quickly. Policosanol has been shown to halt cell overgrowth similar to that of statin drugs.

Animal studies have shown that Policosanol stops the formation of lesions in arteries. One study followed rabbits that were fed a high-cholesterol diet. Researchers found that in "most policosanol-treated animals, atherosclerotic lesions were not present." In other words, it decreases the plaque buildup in the artery walls.

Policosanol has been shown to have a potent antioxidant effect on LDL cholesterol, which re-search has shown to start an inflammatory cascade of events that leads to the development of plaque in the arteries when oxidized.

Policosanol not only lowers the total amount of potentially harmful LDL cholesterol, but it also prevents its oxidation, which is of greater concern than the actual total amount.

Reduces Lipoprotein (a) Levels

As explained in Chapter 1, lipoprotein (a) is a significant heart disease risk marker. Policosanol is one of the few natural substances that have been shown in studies to reduce its levels.

As previously noted, some studies have shown that popular cholesterol-lowering drugs such as Mevacor and Zocor may actually increase the levels of lipoprotein (a).

CHAPTER 3

THE SCIENCE BEHIND POLICOSANOL

There is an abundance of nutritional supplements, many of which are accompanied by extravagant health claims. Few, however, can boast the number of studies that have been made on Policosanol. In terms of rigor, the research on this supplement is comparable to that on most of the pharmaceutical medications on the market.

More than 80,000 people have participated in studies on Policosanol and its effect on cardiovascular health. Numerous studies have been done in Cuba where this medicinal product originated. Quality research has also been conducted in North America and countries around the world. Interest in Policosanol yields numerous published studies yearly. A brief sampling follows.

High Cholesterol

Cholesterol is not really the culprit the medical community and media has made it out to be. Even so, very high levels *can* make one more susceptible to heart disease, particularly elevated LDL cholesterol and lipoprotein (a).

A review of placebo-controlled studies in the *American Heart Journal* found that Policosanol lowered total cholesterol by 17 to 21 percent and LDL cholesterol by 21 to 29 percent, as well as raised the good HDL cholesterol by 8 to 15 percent. The *Journal* also reported that daily doses of 10 mg of Policosanol were found to be as equally effective in lowering total or LDL cholesterol as the statin drugs simvastatin or pravastatin.

While Policosanol has not been found to effectively lower triglyceride levels, many other supplements that will be discussed later in this book can be helpful for this, as can lifestyle changes.

Postmenopausal Women and High Cholesterol

The effects of Policosanol on postmenopausal women were found to be quite positive. The women studied had elevated total and LDL cholesterol even though they were on a standard six-week cholesterol-lowering diet. Ten milligrams of policosanol significantly decreased LDL cholesterol (26.7 percent) and total cholesterol (19.5 percent), while raising HDL cholesterol by 7.4 percent. Women receiving a placebo had no significant changes in cholesterol levels.

Protection for Those with Diabetes

Due to elevated insulin and glucose levels, which create an increased likelihood of cholesterol level imbalance, people with diabetes are much more susceptible to heart disease. Studies have found that Policosanol effectively lowers total and LDL cholesterol in people with non-insulin diabetes. Studies have also shown that Policosanol improves HDL cholesterol more effectively in people with diabetes than the statin drug lovastatin.

Stroke Prevention

Policosanol works to reduce high cholesterol levels and other factors, such as lipoprotein (a), that predispose one to blood clots. Like aspirin, Policosanol was shown in one study to reduce the clumping of blood cells known as platelets, which form blood clots. If platelets clump together too easily, one is more susceptible to formation of a clot, which can cause a stroke. The same study found that Policosanol was more effective than the cholesterol-lowering drug pravastatin in reducing platelet clumping in older patients with high cholesterol.

Angina

This condition, characterized by a tightness or squeezing pain in the chest, is caused by a lack of oxygen to the heart tissue, or a spasm of the heart arteries. In a double-blind study, Policosanol was shown to be effective for patients with angina. The use of Policosanol with aspirin was even more effective than using either of these individual therapies by itself.

Intermittent Claudication

This is a condition in which lower leg pain due to insufficient blood flow is experienced. Risk factors for this condition include diabetes, high blood pressure, high cholesterol, and smoking. All of these contribute to atherosclerosis, the buildup of plaque in the arteries. One landmark study demonstrated that 20 mg a day of Polico - sanol reduced lameness and increased the distance a person could walk by 66 percent.

Policosanol versus Statin Drugs

After several reports in the last few years of serious toxicity that highly publicized cholesterol-lowering statin drugs may cause, consumers are seeking natural alternatives to these medications. One example is the drug Baychol. After a long history of use, it was withdrawn because it was shown to have serious side effects, including liver damage. More than thirty-one people died from its use in the United States before it was taken off the market.

    One of my patients was on this medication

before he came to consult with me. He suffered from fatigue and muscle weakness. After discontinuing the Baychol and substituting Policosanol, his problems went away within two weeks.

The statin drugs are considered conventional medicine's gold standard for cholesterol-lowering medication. Common examples include simivastatin (Zocor) and lovastatin (Mevacor). Policosanol can more than hold its own against these drugs. While they have similar results in lowering LDL and total cholesterol, Policosanol has a better overall effect on elevating the good HDL. A 1999 study, published in the *International Journal of Clinical Pharmacology*, which compared Policosanol with lovastatin, found that only Policosanol significantly elevated HDL levels.

One comparison study found that 10 mg of Policosanol reduced LDL by 24 percent as compared with 22 percent for lovastatin (Mevacor) at 20 mg, and 15 percent for simvastatin (Zocor) at 10 mg. Other studies have found similar results.

Studies in which Policosanol has been combined with cholesterol-lowering drugs to enhance their cholesterol-reducing effects have also been done.

Another advantage of Policosanol is that it does not deplete the body of coenzyme Q_{10}, a critical nutrient for cardiovascular health. A 1993 study in the *Journal of Clinical Pharmacology* found that the use of statin drugs such as pravastatin and simavastatin reduced CoQ_{10} levels by an average of 40 percent after three months of use. Several other studies have also found that CoQ_{10} levels are lowered by the use of these cholesterol-lowering drugs.

Supplementing Policosanol for Optimal Results

Every person is unique and a therapeutic trial of

Policosanol is required to see how it will benefit the individual user. Most positive human studies have used a dosage of 10–20 mg of Policosanol daily. To lower cholesterol and raise the good HDL cholesterol, it is recommended that one start with 10 mg of Policosanol with the evening meal. Your doctor should then order blood work two to three months after beginning supplementation to check your cardiovascular risk markers. If the response is not positive, then the dose should be doubled to 20 mg and testing repeated within two to three months' time.

Some persons may find that even 5 mg per day is enough to achieve a therapeutic response from Policosanol.

Bear in mind that Policosanol does not significantly lower triglyceride levels. If these are elevated, you may find benefit from dietary and lifestyle modifications, as well as other supplements described later in this book, such as fish oil, niacin, pantethine, and garlic.

Using Policosanol with Other Medications and Supplements

One of the unique features of Policosanol is that it does not appear to interfere with the liver's metabolism of drugs. No problems have been found with interactions between Policosanol and heart medications. This includes blood thinners and beta-blockers. In addition, in clinical trials in which Policosanol was given to people taking calcium antagonists, diuretics, vasodilators, non-steroidal anti-inflammatory drugs, meprobamate, thyroid hormones, digoxin, anticoagulants, ulcer drugs, neuroleptics, antidepressants, or anti-anxiety drugs, no problems occurred.

Studies also have found Policosanol to be safe when combined with aspirin, statin cholesterol-lowering medications, and blood pressure med -

icines. It may even enhance the effects of pro-
pranolol, a drug used to lower blood pressure.

Policosanol appears to work synergistically
with many nutritional supplements used to lower
cholesterol. Many doctors and practitioners use
it along with other favorable supplements to
enhance cardiovascular health, such as antioxidants (vitamin A, C, E, and others); essential fatty
acids, including flaxseed or fish oil; and garlic.

Before starting any medication or supplement
program, a doctor should be consulted. The
same rule holds for Policosanol. If you are on
cholesterol-lowering medication, your doctor may
reduce the dosage or even recommend eliminat-
ing it once you have been using Policosanol for
six weeks or longer.

Safety and Toxicity

With any supplement or medication one takes, it
is important to consider the potential for toxicity
and overall safety rating. Fortunately, numerous
human and animal studies confirm that Policosanol is extremely safe. Studies
done with rats given 1,724 times
the regular human dose of
Policosanol found no toxicity.

In one study, the tolerability
of Policosanol was assessed in
more than 27,000 patients. All
of these patients were treated
for at least one month. Only
eighty-six patients (0.31 percent) reported any
adverse effects, the most frequent of which was
weight loss. Twenty-two (0.08 percent) discontinued treatment because of presumed side effects.

Interestingly, placebo-controlled trials found
that side effects from using a placebo were more
common than for Policosanol. The placebo group
and the Policosanol group were equal in reports

Placebo
A "sugar pill"
or other inactive
substance that helps
researchers determine
the effects of a drug
or substance being
tested.

of abdominal pain. It was also found that serious coronary events were fewer in those using Policosanol, compared with those taking a placebo.

Who Should Not Use Policosanol

Although Policosanol did not cause infertility or birth defects in animal studies, it should not be used by pregnant women. This is because, for obvious ethical reasons, human studies have not been done with pregnant women. Secondly, fetal development requires cholesterol and its metabolites, and any agent that restricts this important metabolic factor should be restricted during pregnancy. Also, since Policosanol has not been well studied in this area, breast-feeding mothers should avoid taking Policosanol.

While extremely high cholesterol levels can occur in children, the safe use of Policosanol by children has not been established.

PREVENTING AND TREATING HEART DISEASE

The days of a low-fat, high-carbohydrate diet to prevent and treat heart disease are over as far as nutrition-oriented doctors are concerned. This long-held approach by most cardiologists is fast losing credibility. We know that close to one-fourth of the population is genetically incompatible with this type of diet. Instead, a different dietary approach that takes into account a variety of factors is optimal for heart health. I recommend you follow the dietary recommendations described in this chapter in addition to consulting with a doctor who is trained in nutrition and healthy lifestyle choices. This knowledge will help you optimize your cardiovascular health.

Nutrition-Oriented Doctors
Doctors who place an emphasis on the role of nutrition with their patients.

Power of a Heart-Healthy Diet

What you eat will, to a large extent, determine the health of your heart, arteries, and every other organ in your body. The problem is that people are not too sure what qualifies as a heart-healthy diet. Trendy diets exploited by the media and food industry confuse people so much that as time passes they do not know what to believe. Don't worry about the diet trends that come and go. As with many things in life, it all comes back to doing the basics correctly.

Following are some of the key precepts of a heart-healthy diet. Most people who incorporate these recommendations into their dietary habits will experience a profound effect on their cardio-vascular and overall health.

If your diet is not very healthy right now, please try not to be overwhelmed by all the information being presented. Instead, slowly incorporate these ideas over time. As you feel better from following these recommendations, your confidence in this approach will increase. As in the story of the tortoise and the hare, slow and steady wins the race!

Love Those Veggies

One way or another, we all need to get more vegetables in our diet. While many of us struggle to get a couple of servings of vegetables a day, some experts now recommend getting closer to nine servings daily! Nine servings is a lot, even for the most radical of health food enthusiasts. But the point is that most people would benefit from additional vegetables in their diet.

Vegetables are healthy for the heart in many ways. First of all, they are our best source of fiber. There are two main types of fiber, which are distinguished by how they react to water. Both types are good for you.

Fiber
The indigest-ible portion of plants.

Insoluble fiber cannot dissolve in water and acts as a bulking agent to carry waste products from your digestive tract. A good example is wheat bran.

Soluble fiber (which does dissolve in water) binds cholesterol as it passes through the digestive tract. A great example is oat bran, which has been shown in more than twenty scientific studies to reduce total and LDL cholesterol levels when consumed daily. One bowl of oatmeal daily can lower cholesterol levels between 8 and 23 percent in just three weeks. Pectin, which is found in apple skins, is another great example of soluble fiber that can lower cholesterol. Foods containing both types of fiber should be consumed on a daily basis.

One simple technique I use with patients to get more heart-healthy fiber in the diet is to have them eat a salad or large serving of vegetables with both lunch and dinner. Then, for breakfast, they choose between oatmeal and/or a protein shake combined with a quarter cup of ground flaxseeds. Ground flaxseeds provide a lot of fiber and have been shown to improve cholesterol levels. They also contain a high amount of omega-3 fatty acids, which have been shown to reduce inflammation.

Consume Fats That Heal

One of the biggest problems with the American diet is the type of fat we eat. People are too concerned with limiting their total fat intake. The real issue is that most Americans need to decrease their intake of "bad" fats and increase their intake of "healthy" fats.

Avoid Saturated Fats and Fake Fats

Saturated fats are solid at room temperature. Examples include animal fats such as lard, beef, milk, and cheese. Most people need to decrease the amount of saturated fat in the diet. Too much saturated fat contributes to elevated cholesterol levels. More important, too much saturated fat contributes to an increased inflammatory response in the body.

Saturated fat
A fat that has a carbon molecule saturated with hydrogen molecules.

Other fats to stay away from or limit in the diet include hydrogenated fats. In these fake fats, unsaturated oil has had hydrogen atoms artificially added. This makes margarine solid or semi-solid at room temperature. This type of hydrogenated fat raises LDL levels and lowers the protective HDL cholesterol.

Unsaturated fats, such as those found in flax-seed oil, are healthier for the body.

Get the Right Balance of Fats

Your cells need a balance of essential fatty acids, which the body cannot make on its own. This means that they must be consumed in the diet or taken as a supplement. Essential fatty acids include omega-6 fatty acids, such as corn and safflower oil. However, the majority of our population consumes far too many omega-6 fatty acids (from vegetable cooking oils used in frying and processed foods) and not enough omega-3 fatty acids, found in fish, flaxseeds, and some vegetables. The commercial processing of fats and oils has created an "essential fatty acid crisis" for industrialized nations. These synthetic, rancid fats not only displace "good fats" in the body but they also have toxic effects on the immune, nervous, and cardiovascular systems.

Essential Fatty Acids
Fats the body needs to sustain life.

Many experts feel that the optimal ratio of omega-6 to omega-3 fatty acids is 4:1. Most people consume a ratio closer to 20:1! Society has been on a low-fat diet kick for decades now and more people are overweight than ever before. In addition, diseases related to essential fatty acid deficiency continue to rise. Essential fatty acids influence the passage of nutrients and information that comes into a cell, and the elimination of toxic waste products. As you can see, they are critical for a healthy cardiovascular system. Among other diseases, a deficiency of essential fatty acids contributes to heart disease.

Get Fishy

Several studies have shown that the consumption of cold-water fish such as salmon and halibut provide powerful omega-3 fatty acids for the heart. Interestingly, these omega-3 fatty acids found in fish reduce inflammation in the blood vessels and act as natural blood thinners to prevent stroke and heart attack. Fish also help improve the body's utilization of insulin. Remember that an elevated insulin level is a risk marker for heart disease.

Healing Oils

Healthy oils such as extra-virgin olive oil should be consumed on a regular basis. Olive oil is a great source of omega-9 fatty acids. Although omega-9 fatty acids are not considered essential fatty acids, they play an important role in our health. For example, studies have shown that those who consume olive oil on a regular basis tend to have lower blood pressure. Choose extra-virgin, organic olive oil, as this is the purest form available.

In addition, I highly recommend flaxseed oil be used regularly for a healthy cardiovascular system. Flaxseed oil is a great source of omega-3 fatty acids. It makes an excellent addition to a salad dressing, or can blend in well with a homemade "smoothie." You should avoid heating oils above 325°F as they become oxidized.

Simple Sugars: Enemies of the Heart

It is indisputable that one of the biggest enemies to a healthy heart is the "standard American diet." High amounts of simple sugars, saturated fats, processed foods, and oils accelerate the development of heart disease. These foods, which exemplify the fast food menu of Americans today, are the recipe for a premature heart attack.

"Processed carbohydrates" is really another way of saying "simple sugars." Refined flours that make up most of the breads, cereals, pastries, and pastas people eat have been stripped of their fiber and nutrients. As a result, these foods cause blood sugar levels to soar, and in response to this increase in blood sugar, the hormone known as insulin spikes. This sets up a process: the body stores the blood sugar as fat, elevating cholesterol and other risk factors for heart disease. Underlying this process is inflammation within the cardiovascular system, which these refined carbohydrates cause.

The best way to avoid processed carbohydrates is to avoid packaged food as much as possible. Try to eat food in its natural state by creating as many meals as you can at home from fresh, unprocessed ingredients.

The carbohydrates you do eat should be complex carbohydrates. Examples include low glycemic vegetables such as broccoli, asparagus, spinach, cabbage, legumes, lentils, soy, chickpeas, and onions. High-fiber pastas made from spelt or amaranth is preferable over semolina flour pasta that is refined. Please note that some people do not do well with any type of grain. Some have sensitivity to or are allergic to wheat and other gluten-containing grains. Such allergies may cause digestive and blood sugar problems that can worsen inflammation in the arteries. If you suspect that you have this problem, consult with a nutrition-oriented doctor to investigate this further.

Complex Carbohydrates
Long chains of sugars that release sugars slowly into the body.

Eat Quality Protein

Good protein sources include cold-water fish such as salmon, mackerel, sardines, and halibut.

Organic eggs are also good, as are legumes and soy products such as tofu, soymilk, and tempeh.

Drink Cleaner Water

Clean drinking water is of enormous importance to the health of your heart and cardiovascular system. More than half of our entire body weight is composed of water.

As a general rule, it's best that you not rely on your local tap water as your primary source of drinking water. The high chlorine content common in nearly all municipal water systems may contribute to heart disease and other maladies. Also, regular tap water carries a risk of parasitic infection.

Certified water purification systems that also remove lead, mercury, arsenic, cadmium, and other toxic elements that cause cardiovascular damage through free-radical formation are best. If possible, I recommend purchasing or renting a reverse osmosis system for your home. As a first step, a carbon-filter system attached to your drinking faucet will still go a long way in improving the quality of your water.

Can the Caffeine

Caffeine may give you a jolt of energy, but it also depletes the heart of magnesium, calcium, and other valuable minerals required for energy production within the heart cells. Deficiencies of these minerals can also contribute to high blood pressure. Forego the latte and switch to organic green tea (half the amount of caffeine) and other herbal teas. Also, try to incorporate fresh vegetable and fruit juices into your diet. These juices are abundant in a variety of minerals.

Add Spice to Your Life

I highly recommend that you consume more flavorful herbs and spices on a regular basis. Many, such as cayenne, basil, rosemary, garlic, onions, and oregano, provide excellent antioxidant and nutritional support for the cardiovascular system.

Onions, for example, have been shown in studies to lower cholesterol and triglycerides. They also are a great source of vitamin C and aid the body in detoxification. Oregano has potent antimicrobial effects and may help prevent chronic infections in the body. Cayenne is not only a strong antioxidant, but also helps to thin the blood for improved circulation. Rosemary has some of the most potent antioxidants known. Like onions, it also supports the liver in effective detoxification.

These herbs and spices are excellent enhancements to flavor your meals, and can be a satisfying alternative to salt.

A Healthy Heart Needs Exercise

Perhaps the easiest way to reduce your risk of heart disease is to get on a regular exercise regimen. Exercise has a wide range of benefits to the cardiovascular system. It has been shown to lower cholesterol levels, raise the good HDL cholesterol, improve insulin sensitivity, and reduce blood pressure. Also, exercise has been shown to reduce depression and improve sleep—both of which also benefit the heart. Lastly, exercise also burns calories. Losing weight is an excellent way you can take a burden off your heart. Let's face it, no single supplement or food can beat all the heart-healthy benefits you can get from exercise.

Doing some aerobic exercise only three days a week will provide a beneficial effect on the cardiovascular system. The Nurses Health Study, which analyzed the histories of more than 72,000 women, found that even brisk walking for three hours per week cut the risk of cardiovascular disease by a whopping 40 percent!

The biggest dilemma people frequently have when it comes to exercise is choosing the right exercise program. I have a simple solution: choose an exercise or combination of exercises that you truly enjoy. The reality is that when a person picks an exercise program they really like, the odds are better that they will be motivated to stay with it. On the other hand, if you feel you are forcing yourself to endure a particular exercise regimen that you really don't have any passion for, you most likely won't stick with it.

In general, I recommend starting with an exercise program that includes aerobic activities such as walking, biking, swimming, or some sport or activity that keeps you moving continuously for twenty minutes or longer. Over time, it is also good to incorporate some resistance training, such as light weight lifting, into your program.

You may be one of those who require a trainer to keep you on track. That's okay. Most fitness clubs offer plenty of assistance in helping you design an exercise program to meet your goals.

It is recommended that you consult with your doctor first before starting any exercise program. This is especially important if you have any medical condition or have not exercised in a long time.

CHAPTER 5

HEART-HEALTHY NUTRIENTS

Nature has provided numerous vitamins and mineral supplements that guard against the causes of heart disease in a variety of ways. Each of the nutrients discussed in this chapter has its own unique benefit(s) in reducing the risk factors associated with cardiovascular disease. The key is to use the right combination and amounts when supplementing these safe and effective nutrients.

Niacin

One of the oldest therapies for treating high cholesterol levels is vitamin B_3, commonly referred to as niacin. Vitamin B_3 has been shown in several studies to lower total and LDL cholesterol, tri glycerides, and fibrinogen, as well as decrease lipoprotein (a). Simultaneously, it increases the good HDL cholesterol.

As mentioned in Chapter 1, elevated Lp(a) is an independent risk factor for cardiovascular disease. Niacin has been shown to be a very effective treatment for those with elevated Lp(a) and low HDL cholesterol. If you have imbalances with both of these markers, niacin is an excellent choice that can help you achieve measurable improvements in both markers. Surprisingly, even though many studies have shown it to be as effective as many pharmaceutical medications, and at a fraction of the cost, it is rarely prescribed by physicians.

The relationship of niacin to elevated cholesterol and triglyceride levels has been the focus of many studies. Some studies have done head-to-head comparisons between niacin and cholesterol-lowering medications. One study, for example, compared the effectiveness of niacin with the statin drug lovastatin. This study looked at the effects of these two treatments on 136 patients with elevated LDL cholesterol levels. Lovastatin had a greater benefit in reducing LDL levels while niacin was more effective in elevating HDL cholesterol. Niacin was also more effective in lowering Lp(a). In fact, niacin reduced Lp(a) by 35 percent, while lovastatin had no effect.

Niacin also has proven itself to be a valuable supplement for people with diabetes, and the elevation of cardiovascular markers that generally accompany this disease.

Several studies have also shown that niacin enhances the cholesterol-reducing effect of several pharmaceutical cholesterol-lowering medications. And, it works quite well in conjunction with a variety of natural cholesterol-lowering supplements.

The Other Niacin

In the health food industry "niacin" generally refers to Vitamin B_3. However, there is a variant of niacin known as niacinamide. Niacinamide is used therapeutically for conditions such as osteoarthritis and diabetes, not for cholesterol.

Avoid the "Flush"

Some people experience a flushing reaction fifteen to thirty minutes after taking niacin. Symptoms often include a warming sensation followed by perspiring and reddening of the skin. In some cases, this may be accompanied by anxiety and/

or digestive upset. Sensitivity reactions such as these are not life threatening, but still are completely avoidable with a readily available non-flush form known as inositol hexaniacinate. Bottles generally will be labeled "No-flush Niacin" or "Flush Free Niacin." The cost is slightly higher, but this is the type of niacin that I, as well as most natural healthcare practitioners, recommend.

No Flush Niacin

A type of niacin known as Inositol hexaniacinate that does not cause the flushing of the skin that some people experience with regular niacin.

Dosage

I recommend starting with 1,500 mg daily for those with mild to moderate cholesterol elevations and working up to 3,000 mg daily for those with severely elevated cholesterol levels.

Food Sources

Good sources of niacin include brewer's yeast, eggs, fish, peanuts, legumes, whole grains, and organ meats.

Other B Vitamins

All of the B vitamins are important for your cardiovascular and overall health. However, there are three in particular that researchers have found to be important for a healthy heart and circulatory system. These three include vitamin B_{12}, folic acid, and vitamin B_6.

In Chapter 1, I explained that elevated levels of the blood marker homocysteine are much more predictive of heart disease than is high cholesterol. This byproduct of protein metabolism is a significant risk factor for a heart attack or stroke. Many people (5 to 10 percent of the population) have a genetic defect that causes elevated homocysteine levels; for them, diet has little to do with it. In others, these levels can creep up as a result of a high animal protein diet or low thyroid function.

Have your doctor order a blood test that measures homocysteine levels. If your levels are elevated, there is no need to panic. Simply supplementing with additional vitamin B_{12}, folic acid, and vitamin B_6 can get the levels down to normal. For only about ten dollars a month, you can prevent a future major cardiovascular problem by supplementing with these nontoxic B vitamins. Researchers have estimated that if we all supplemented with folic acid alone, it would save 20,000 to 50,000 premature deaths annually from heart attack in the United States.

Dosage

By following your homocysteine levels with blood tests, your doctor can help determine the optimal dosage of these B vitamins. Following is a general daily guideline for those with elevated homocysteine levels:

Vitamin B_{12}:	800–2,000 mcg daily
Folic acid:	1–10 mg daily
Vitamin B_6:	20–100 mg daily

It is now common to find "homocysteine formulas" that contain high dosages of these B vitamins. This often eliminates the need to buy each individually.

Vitamin E

There are few supplements that have as much scientific research behind them with regard to efficacy in reducing the risk of heart disease as vitamin E. It has not only been shown to effectively prevent heart disease, but can also benefit those with existing cardiovascular disease. So revered is this vitamin that a poll of cardiologists found that 44 percent use it themselves for the prevention of heart disease.

Vitamin E is the body's most important fat-soluble antioxidant. As an antioxidant, it prevents cholesterol (specifically LDL cholesterol) from becoming oxidized. In so doing, it ultimately prevents inflammation of the arteries and the plaque buildup that leads to hardening of the arteries. Vitamin E also has a blood-thinning effect so that deadly blood clots do not form as easily. When used consistently, vitamin E works to prevent strokes and heart attacks from occurring.

Protects Against the Fast Food Diet

A 1997 study done at the University of Maryland caught the attention of doctors and the health food community. Cardiologist Gary Plotnick and his associates looked at the effect of supplemental vitamin E and vitamin C on people eating a high-fat meal.

In this study, twenty healthy volunteers between the ages of twenty-four and fifty-four ate a high-fat breakfast consisting of eggs, sausage, hash browns, and a roll. As expected, ultrasound measurements, which assess blood flow, found that this meal negatively affected blood flow. Then, on another day, the same people took 800 IU of vitamin E and 1,000 mg of vitamin C before consuming an identical breakfast. This time, the measurements of their blood flow were normal. This benefit was found to last for six hours.

Another study, published in the *American Journal of Preventive Medicine* in 2001, found similar benefits.

Helpful for Heart Disease

In 1996, the Cambridge Heart Study was noted as one of the most important medical accomplishments. This study looked at the effect of vitamin E on 2,000 people who had heart disease. It found that those who took between 400 and 800 IU of vitamin E had a 77 percent decrease in cardiovascular disease over a year's time!

Another study, sponsored by the National Institute of Aging, followed more than 11,000 seniors for nine years. Researchers found that those seniors who supplemented with 400 IU of vitamin E daily had a 41 percent reduction in heart disease.

And finally, one of the studies I most often cite during lectures is the Nurses Health Study. In this study, which involved 87,000 women, researchers reported that those who took vitamin E for two years or more had a 41 percent reduction in the risk of heart disease.

There are many more studies I could cite that have scientifically validated the cardiovascular benefits of vitamin E. This common vitamin is a powerful antioxidant and protector of the heart. What a safe and inexpensive way to prevent the deadly effects of heart disease.

The Vitamin E Family

Vitamin E has more than one form. Most of the focus on vitamin E in the past has been on one form known as d-alpha tocopherol. This is the "natural" form of vitamin E that has been recommended by nutrition-oriented physicians for decades. While d-alpha tocopherol is responsible for most of the activity of vitamin E, we must recognize that there are also three other tocopherols in the vitamin E family. These include beta, gamma, and delta tocopherols. Research is finding that each of these individual tocopherols has its own unique antioxidant properties.

Natural Vitamin E

Vitamin E, as it is found in nature, is labeled as d-alpha tocopherol on supplement containers.

Vitamin E supplements are now available that are labeled "mixed vitamin E." I prefer this type because it provides the user with the full spectrum of antioxidant properties of all the tocopherols in one formula.

More Vitamin E Benefits

There is more to the vitamin E story than just the family of tocopherols. Another important group of compounds is also part of the vitamin E family. These are tocotrienols. There are four different forms of tocotrienols. These compounds also have potent antioxidant activity, and unlike the tocopherols, they have been shown to be effective in reducing cholesterol levels. While they can be found as part of a comprehensive vitamin E complex (along with tocopherols), tocotrienols really need to be taken as a separate supplement in order to get an amount great enough to lower cholesterol.

Dosage

For most people, I recommend 400 IU of natural

Carotid Stenosis & Tocotrienol

Tocotrienol supplements may be your best option to surgery for *carotid stenosis* (buildup of plaque that narrows the carotid arteries and restricts blood flow to the brain). The surgery for carotid stenosis is quite dangerous with a 1 in 10 risk of stroke and death. A four-year study looked at people with severe carotid stenosis who were given either tocotrienols or a placebo. Ultrasound analysis showed that 94 percent of those taking tocotrienols improved or stabilized. The condition of half of those given a placebo worsened, while that of the other half in the placebo group remained the same.

vitamin E to be taken daily. Keep in mind that many quality high-potency multivitamins contain this much vitamin E. Vitamin E is a fat-soluble vitamin. This means that it requires some fat for optimal absorption so it is best taken with a meal.

For those who are exposed to higher than average environmental pollution (smoke, for instance), or those who for some reason are consuming an unhealthy diet of fast foods, I recommend taking a dosage of 800 IU daily.

If you are using vitamin E to reduce cholesterol levels, you should use a tocotrienols complex. A dosage of 100–400 mg may be required to lower total and LDL cholesterol.

Cheaper synthetic versions of vitamin E are available on the market. They are labeled as dl-alpha tocopherol. I tell patients that if there is an "l" in it then "leave" it alone. Natural vitamin E such as d-alpha tocopherol or the mixed vitamin E is much better, and studies show these are absorbed twice as efficiently as synthetic vitamin E.

The key to getting all the cardiovascular benefits of vitamin E is to consume foods rich in this nutrient and to take vitamin E supplements on a regular basis. The benefits of vitamin E are achieved over months and years, not days and weeks.

Safety

Vitamin E has an excellent safety record. The major caution for vitamin E is for those on blood-thinning medications such as Coumadin. If you are taking blood-thinning medications, consult with your physician before beginning supplementation with vitamin E. Most people can take a lower dosage of 200–400 IU of vitamin E while on these medications if properly monitored by their doctor.

Vitamin E can also improve glucose tolerance in some people with diabetes. I recommend that those on diabetic medications consult with their doctor before using more than 400 IU of vitamin E, as their medication dosages may need to be decreased over time.

Food Sources

Vitamin E occurs naturally in the fats of vegetables. Wheat-germ oil, whole grains, nuts, seeds, legumes, and dark-green leafy vegetables are good sources.

Vitamin C

Many people know vitamin C as the main nutrient that supports the immune system to fight colds and flu. Well, vitamin C not only helps prevent infections, but it also is a key nutrient for the heart. Many population studies demonstrate that vitamin C reduces the risk of death from strokes and heart attacks.

Vitamin C is the body's most important water-soluble antioxidant. It prevents cholesterol, especially LDL cholesterol, from becoming oxidized.

Because our bodies cannot manufacture it, we must get vitamin C from our diet or as a supplement.

Improves Cholesterol Levels

Numerous studies have shown that vitamin C significantly reduces the risk of dying from heart disease. Vitamin C can reduce total and LDL cholesterol levels. One of the mechanisms for this benefit is that vitamin C is involved in the formation of bile salts. Bile is produced by the liver and stored and released by the gallbladder for the digestion of fats. Cholesterol is converted into bile salts and vitamin C enhances this process, thus reducing cholesterol levels.

One of the better-designed studies showed a correlation between the higher the vitamin C content of blood, the lower the total cholesterol and triglyceride levels. This same study also showed a very positive elevation in HDL levels. Another impressive study found that 3 grams of vitamin C taken on a daily basis decreased cholesterol levels by 18 percent and triglycerides by 12 percent in three weeks.

One of vitamin C's many functions is improving the strength and elasticity of blood vessel walls. Vitamin C is a necessary cofactor in the production of collagen. Collagen is a protein substance that holds connective tissue together, including that of blood vessels.

It was postulated by Nobel laureate Linus Pauling that a vitamin C deficiency increases the likelihood that blood vessel walls will be weaker and thinner. As a result, damage can occur to weakened spots in the blood vessel walls, which then are patched by the body with plaque formation. However, he postulated, this dangerous sequence can be prevented or treated with extra supplementation of vitamin C.

For Smokers

It is a well-known fact that smokers have a vastly increased risk for heart disease. Toxic byproducts of tobacco smoke greatly increase the amount of free radicals in the body. As a result, cholesterol becomes oxidized much more quickly. While it makes most sense just to quit smoking completely, all smokers should consider vitamin C supplementation.

One study found that, in smokers, vitamin C reduced aggregation of platelets, the sticky substances that promote clotting of the blood. This same benefit was also found in nonsmokers who supplemented vitamin C.

High Blood Pressure

Several population and clinical studies show that the higher a person's vitamin C levels are the lower the blood pressure will be. Researchers at the Boston University School of Medicine and the Linus Pauling Institute at Oregon State University conducted a study in which forty-five patients were given either 500 mg of vitamin C or a placebo each day. After one month, those who took the vitamin C had a 9 percent drop in total blood pressure. Those on the placebo had no change. Vitamin C had no effect on those who had normal blood pressure.

Circulation, Stroke, and Angina

Elevated blood pressure is a significant risk factor for stroke. A ten-year study involving almost 2,500 men found that a low blood level of vitamin C was associated with increased risk of stroke. This was especially true among men who were overweight and had high blood pressure.

Vitamin C has been shown to be helpful for patients with angina (chest pain). By acting as an antioxidant, vitamin C helps maintain the body's levels of nitric oxide (NO), a natural chemical messenger in the body that acts to relax blood vessels. This activity promotes healthy circulation and lowers the pressure inside blood vessels.

Like vitamin E, vitamin C has been shown to

Vitamin C and Bypass Surgery

Vitamin C supplementation appears to be very important after heart surgery. One hospital study found vitamin C status decreased by 70 percent within twenty-four hours after coronary bypass surgery. In most patients, this deficiency lasted up to two weeks after the initial surgery.

maintain healthy circulation after a high-fat meal. A recent cardiology study of patients with coronary heart disease found this benefit to be quite significant.

Dosage

For the general prevention of heart disease, I recommend between 500 and 1,000 mg of vitamin C daily. For those with existing heart disease, I prefer a dosage of 2,000–3,000 mg daily, or higher if your nutrition-oriented doctor so recommends.

There are several different forms of vitamin C. I usually recommend that my patients use buffered vitamin C as it reduces the likelihood of digestive irritation. Buffered vitamin C is a product that binds vitamin C to a mineral salt, such as calcium ascorbate or sodium ascorbate.

Safety

Contrary to some reports you may hear in the media, the safety record of vitamin C is excellent. The most common side effect is digestive upset, which may be alleviated by taking vitamin C with food or by using buffered vitamin C. In addition, some people may experience diarrhea if they are taking too high a dosage.

> **Buffered Vitamin C**
> *Vitamin C that is attached to a mineral salt to reduce acidity reactions such as heartburn.*

Food Sources

Fruits and vegetables are excellent sources of vitamin C. Especially good examples are citrus fruits, tomatoes, peppers, dark-green leafy vegetables, broccoli, kale, strawberries, and potatoes.

Pantethine

Pantethine is a metabolite of vitamin B_5 (pantothenic acid). This vitamin supplement has been shown in several studies to reduce triglycerides and LDL cholesterol, while simultaneously in - creasing the helpful HDL cholesterol. Pantethine works by slowing the production of cholesterol in the liver and by increasing the rate of fat metabolism.

This nutrient has been used for the past thirty years in Japan as a pharmaceutical agent to im- prove cholesterol levels. Pantethine is sold as a supplement in the United States and is available in most health food stores and pharmacies.

Support for Those with Diabetes

Pantethine has proven to be very effective for diabetic patients. It is common for diabetics to have elevated cholesterol and triglyceride levels. For example, in one study, diabetic patients were given 600 mg of pantethine for three months and then 1,200 mg for an additional six months. Supplementation of pantethine was shown to significantly reduce triglyceride and total choles- terol levels. Other studies have shown pantethine to be quite effective as a supplement for diabet- ic patients receiving dialysis.

Dosage

The typical dosage of pantethine to help balance lipid levels is 600–900 mg daily. It is best taken in two to three separate doses.

Safety

Research over the past thirty years on pantethine has found no significant adverse effects.

Carnitine

Carnitine is a natural substance that is utilized within the cells to burn fat for energy production. Meat and dairy products are the major food sources of this vitaminlike substance. In addition, your body can manufacture carnitine from the amino acid lysine.

Studies have shown that carnitine reduces total cholesterol and triglyceride levels and raises HDL cholesterol. Using carnitine, one can expe - rience up to a 25 percent decrease in triglyceride levels. Carnitine is of special value in reducing cholesterol levels for those with kidney disease who are receiving hemodialysis.

Carnitine provides a number of benefits to the heart. Numerous studies have confirmed its ame- lioration of such conditions as angina, arrhyth- mia, and congestive heart failure.

Dosage

The recommended dosage is 1,500–4,000 mg daily taken in divided doses. The proper form to use as a supplement is L-carnitine.

Safety

L-carnitine is a very safe supplement. A small per- centage of people may experi- ence digestive upset, which may be resolved by taking it along with a meal. Patients who are on hemodialysis should supplement L-carnitine only under the super- vision of a physician.

Hemodialysis
Regular blood filtration by a machine, undergone by persons with kidney disease.

Coenzyme Q₁₀

One of the most important nutrients for the heart is coenzyme Q_{10}, also referred to as CoQ_{10}. Like carnitine, CoQ_{10}, as it is most often called, is essential for energy production within heart cells, as well as within the rest of the body's cells. It helps the heart to beat with strong, regular series of rhythmical contractions. As a result, blood flow improves throughout the circulatory system and tissues fill with vital oxygen.

Food sources of CoQ_{10} include meat, fish, and nuts. The body also manufactures CoQ_{10} from the amino acid tyrosine.

Perhaps no other nutrient provides as many benefits for the heart and cardiovascular system as CoQ_{10}. Nutrition-oriented doctors use CoQ_{10} to treat angina, heart arrhythmia, cardiomyopathy, congestive heart failure, mitral valve prolapse, and high blood pressure. CoQ_{10} is a potent antioxidant that helps prevent the oxidation of cholesterol.

CoQ_{10} and Statin Drugs

CoQ_{10} is a very important nutrient to supplement with if you are currently taking a cholesterol-lowering "statin" drug. This class of popular cholesterol-lowering medications work by inhibiting an enzyme in the liver that produces cholesterol. This same enzyme is involved in the synthesis of CoQ_{10}. Examples of "statin" medications that may deplete CoQ_{10} include Zocor, Mevacor, and Pravachol. If you are taking one of these medications, it is recommended that you supplement with 100 mg of CoQ_{10} daily to prevent a deficiency.

Dosage

I recommend that those with elevated cholesterol levels take 50–100 mg of CoQ_{10} daily. If you are currently using a "statin" cholesterol-lowering drug make sure to take 100 mg daily. Higher dosages of up to 500 mg daily are used by nutrition-oriented doctors for those with serious heart disease.

Safety

CoQ_{10} is very safe. It has a mild blood-thinning

effect, so those on blood-thinning medications, such as Coumadin, should be monitored by their physician while using CoQ_{10}.

Magnesium

After potassium, magnesium is the second most abundant mineral in the body's cells. It is essential for a healthy heart and cardiovascular system. It is involved in more than 300 enzymatic reactions in the body. This includes energy production, heart contraction, and the relaxation of blood vessels.

Studies have shown that many people who have heart attacks have low magnesium levels. This is at least partly due to the fact that magnesium helps regulate heart rhythm, as well as helps dilate coronary arteries to optimize oxygenation of heart tissue. Along with carnitine and CoQ_{10}, magnesium should be considered essential for those with congestive heart failure, mitral valve prolapse, and high blood pressure.

One of the main benefits of magnesium is that it acts as a smooth muscle relaxer. Since blood vessel walls are surrounded by smooth muscle, magnesium helps to dilate the arteries so there can be optimal blood flow. This also translates into lower blood pressure, for which magnesium is especially helpful.

Dosage

The average dosage for supplemental magne - sium is 500 mg daily. Nutrition-oriented doc - tors may use up to 1,000 mg daily and, in some cases, may prescribe intravenous treatments of magnesium.

Safety

Some people may experience diarrhea with higher dosages of magnesium. This can often be avoided by slowly increasing the dose over time or by using forms of magnesium less likely to cause diarrhea such as magnesium glycinate. Those with heart and kidney disease should not use magnesium supplements unless it is under the guidance of a physician.

Food Sources

Magnesium can be found in foods such as whole grains, legumes, nuts, and green leafy vegetables.

Antioxidants

There are numerous other nutritional supplements that are protective for the heart. Among the most important is a whole class of nutrients known as antioxidants.

As discussed in Chapter 1, the main concern with moderate to high levels of cholesterol is the increased amount of oxidation that can occur with these fatty substances. As a result of oxidation, blood vessel inflammation and damage is more likely to occur. Antioxidants from the foods we eat (mainly plant foods) are our primary defense against oxidized cholesterol, which contributes greatly to cardiovascular disease.

Antioxidants
Substances that neutralize or reduce the effects of cell-damaging free radicals.

Dosage

The most practical way to get a full spectrum of antioxidants is to supplement with a high potency multivitamin and mineral formula. This will give you a base of many of the antioxidants. In addition, if the need for extra supplementation is required due to physical illness or higher demand (both smokers and athletes will need more), antioxidant formulas can be used that contain higher levels of the important antioxidants.

Safety

Antioxidant supplements are very safe. Nonetheless, if you are receiving chemotherapy or radiation treatments for cancer, or if you are pregnant or planning to become pregnant, check with your doctor first before using.

Food Sources

Many foods contain high-antioxidant activity. Among the best are fruits such as blueberries, cranberries, grapes, lemons, limes, strawberries, cherries, oranges, tomatoes, and cantaloupe. Many vegetables also contain an array of nature's powerful antioxidants—broccoli, carrots, squash, kale, cauliflower, Brussels sprouts, and dark-green leafy vegetables. Common kitchen herbs, spices, and savory vegetables (onions, garlic) are some of the most powerful antioxidant-containing foods; try using oregano, rosemary, and turmeric to season your dishes. And lastly, teas, such as green and black tea, contain powerful antioxidants known as polyphenols.

Beyond the diet, numerous antioxidants are available in supplement form. Common antioxidant supplements that you will find on the shelves of health food stores and pharmacies include vitamin A, vitamin C, vitamin E, selenium, carotenoids, lipoic acid, coenzyme Q_{10}, zinc, N-acetylcysteine, L-glutathione, Pycnogenol, and grape seed extract.

CHAPTER 6

HEART-HEALTHY HERBAL REMEDIES

A variety of herbal supplements have been used throughout the ages to prevent and treat various cardiovascular problems. In the past decade, scientific research has validated the benefits of many of these herbs.

Hawthorn Berry

One of the true superstars when it comes to herbal remedies that support heart and cardiovascular health is hawthorn berry. Hawthorn has long been used by herbalists and natural doctors in Europe, and it can benefit millions of Americans with angina, coronary artery disease, arrhythmia, congestive heart failure, and high blood pressure. It is an excellent herb to help strengthen and tone the heart muscle.

There are many parts of the hawthorn plant that are used medicinally such as the leaves, flowers, and berries. However, most hawthorn extracts use the berry, which contains a group of flavonoids that support the cardiovascular system.

Flavonoids
A group of plant pigments that are responsible for the color of flowers and fruits.

Flavonoids are effective in relaxing the coronary arteries, facilitating improved blood flow to the heart and cells of the body, and ameliorating high blood pressure.

Angina

The pain of angina may be described as a squeezing sensation of the heart. There may be a number of causes for angina; one of the most common is impeded blood flow, leading to a shortage of oxygen reaching the heart cells. The impeded flow of blood is usually due to coronary artery disease, where plaque has built up in the arteries that feed the heart. Since hawthorne dilates the coronary arteries to improve blood flow and oxygenation of the heart, it is a valuable herb for preventing angina.

In a three-week study, researchers found that hawthorn had a significant effect on blood flow to the heart. Patients who used hawthorn in this study also showed a 25 percent improvement in their ability to tolerate exercise.

Arrhythmia

Hawthorn is commonly used by naturopathic doctors and herbalists to treat non-life-threatening heart arrhythmias. This approach works even better when combined with coenzyme Q_{10}, carnitine, and magnesium supplements.

Congestive Heart Failure

The majority of the research that has been done on hawthorn has focused on its benefit for treating congestive heart failure.

Congestive Heart Failure
A condition in which the heart can no longer pump blood efficiently to meet the demands of the body.

Most cases of congestive heart failure are due to arterio-sclerosis—the buildup of plaque in the heart arteries, or long-standing high blood pressure.

A number of studies have demonstrated the benefit of hawthorn for this serious condition. The German Commission E, the official government agency that evaluates the effectiveness of herbs in Germany, supports the medical use of hawthorn in the treatment of this disease.

In one high-quality study, researchers found that eight weeks of hawthorn supplementation improved heart function and reduced symptoms in people who had a rating of moderate congestive heart failure. In another study, patients supplemented 900 mg daily doses of hawthorn extract. Researchers found the benefit equal to that of commonly used heart medications but without the side effects often found with these pharmaceuticals.

High Blood Pressure

Hawthorn is often the key herbal element found in high blood pressure formulas available in North American health food stores and pharmacies. As it relaxes the artery walls, pressure inside the blood vessels decreases. Several studies have found it effective for those with elevated blood pressure.

Dosage

I recommend using hawthorn extracts standardized to 2.2 percent flavonoids or 18.75 percent procyanidins. The milligram dosage is usually between 500 and 900 mg daily.

Safety

Hawthorn is a very safe supplement and can be used on a long-term basis. Those on hypertension medications such as digitalis, coumadin, and beta-blockers should consult with a physician before starting hawthorn supplementation so that they can be properly monitored.

Garlic

One of the world's most popular food flavorings,

garlic is also one of the most popular and well-studied herbal supplements. To date, more than 200 human studies and 800 animal studies have looked at the many health benefits of garlic.

Numerous studies have shown that garlic lowers total and LDL cholesterol while improving HDL cholesterol. It has also been shown in recent studies to lower homocysteine. In addition, garlic is an herbalist's ally in the fight against high blood pressure, aging coronary arteries, and for promoting circulation by acting as a natural blood thinner. If that is not enough, garlic also has beneficial antioxidant activity.

Lowers Cholesterol and Homocysteine

Several studies have shown that garlic works to reduce cholesterol, triglyceride, and homocysteine levels. In an overview of sixteen garlic studies that involved 952 people, researchers found that garlic lowered total cholesterol by 12 percent after one to three months of use. Many of these studies used dried garlic powder at a daily dosage that ranged between 600 and 900 mg.

Studies have also shown garlic to lower LDL cholesterol and homocysteine. Garlic is one of the few supplements shown to increase the beneficial HDL cholesterol.

Animal studies have shown that garlic inhibits the production of cholesterol by the liver and also enhances the breakdown and excretion of cholesterol.

Aorta
A very large blood vessel that carries oxygenated blood from the heart to the rest of the body.

Improved Artery Elasticity

A 1997 study of garlic's properties came to the conclusion that "garlic intake had a protective effect on the elastic properties of the aorta related to aging in humans."

Stiffening of the aorta makes

this artery more likely to burst. This is a life-threatening event, and high blood pressure and nutritional deficiencies are considered to be underlying causes of stiff arteries.

Reduces Blood Pressure

Garlic is a good herb to use as a food and supplement on a long-term basis for the reduction of mildly elevated blood pressure. Preliminary research has shown that garlic has a relaxant effect on the smooth muscles of the heart and arteries.

Thins the Blood

Human and animal studies have proven that garlic has natural blood-thinning qualities. This may prove to be an effective supplement in the prevention of blood clots and strokes.

Potent Antioxidant

One of garlic's many benefits is that it prevents the oxidation of cholesterol and other fats in the blood. In one study, ten volunteers supplemented with garlic powder tablets for two weeks. Researchers found that there was a 34 percent reduction in the oxidation of blood fats.

Dosage

Garlic supplements come in a variety of forms. Enteric-coated tablets of fresh garlic powder are effective at a dosage of 600–900 mg daily. In addition, aged garlic has also proven to be beneficial for elevated cholesterol and homocysteine levels.

Safety

Garlic has long been considered safe as a food and supplement. Since it has natural blood-thinning properties, it should be used under a doctor's supervision if blood-thinning medications are being taken.

Guggul

The discovery of guggul, a small tree that is native to India and Bangladesh, as the source of a cholesterol-lowering supplement has a fairly unusual history. During the 1960s, an Indian researcher read about the effectiveness of guggul to help with blood fat disorders and obesity in an ancient Ayurvedic medical textbook. Inspired by this ancient information, researchers began animal studies to determine its effect on heart disease. It was discovered that the extract from underneath the tree's bark contains a group of chemicals known as guggulipids that exert an anticholesterol and anti-inflammatory effect.

Early animal studies showed that guggul significantly reduced high cholesterol levels. Subsequent human studies over the past forty years have shown that guggul extract is an effective therapy to reduce cholesterol and triglyceride levels. Current studies show it to be as effective as some cholesterol-lowering drugs.

Guggul stimulates the liver's metabolism of cholesterol. It also improves thyroid function, which affects cholesterol levels. And lastly, it has a natural blood-thinning effect by preventing the clumping of platelets, the cells responsible for blood clotting.

Help for High Cholesterol

Guggul extract has been shown to reduce total cholesterol, LDL, VLDL (very low density lipo - protein, which carries cholesterol in the arteries), and triglyceride levels. As an added bonus, it can increase HDL cholesterol.

A twelve-week study demonstrated that 1,500 mg of guggulipid reduced total cholesterol by an average of 22 percent and triglycerides by 25 percent. Another study of 233 people with elevated cholesterol or triglyceride levels showed that guggulipid worked better than the cholesterol-lowering drug clofibrate. Only those taking guggulipid had an improvement in HDL cholesterol.

Dosage

For the reduction of cholesterol and triglycerides, I recommend a daily total of 1,500 mg of a 5 percent guggulsterone standardized extract. This is equivalent to 75 mg of guggulsterones. The supplement should be taken for at least two months before lipid levels are reevaluated.

Safety

A small percentage of users experience digestive upset from guggul supplementation. It should not be used during pregnancy or by those with heavy uterine bleeding. There are no known harmful drug interactions with guggul.

Ginkgo Biloba

Ginkgo is one of America's most popular herbal supplements. Fossil records show ginkgo to be one of the oldest living species of tree on the planet, and this amazing herb has a history of use that dates back almost 5,000 years in traditional Chinese herbal therapy.

Ginkgo receives a lot of well-deserved attention for its ability to improve memory. However, it also is gaining acceptance as one of the most important herbs for the cardiovascular system. Ginkgo has been shown to have potent positive effects on circulation. It has a mild blood-thinning effect and is thought to help prevent stroke; it works to dilate blood vessels, which improves circulation to all areas of the body; this action helps reduce blood pressure, as well. It also has been shown to provide some of nature's most potent antioxidants.

Medicinal Properties of Ginkgo

During the 1950s, European researchers began investigating the medicinal properties of ginkgo leaves, particularly the beneficial effects on circulation and memory. It has been shown that unique active components in ginkgo account for much of its therapeutic activity.

One of the main active components found in ginkgo are bioflavonoids known as flavone glycosides. These account for ginkgo's powerful antioxidant properties, which, when ingested, help protect the body against the ravages of pollution and other causes of free-radical damage. They also work to strengthen blood vessel walls to make them more resilient against inflammation and rupture.

Other important components are terpene lactones. These lactones enable ginkgo to increase circulation by causing blood vessels to relax and dilate. They also provide potent antioxidant activity to scavenge free radicals, thereby preventing brain and nerve damage. A specific type of terpene lactone known as ginkgolides B is very effective in reducing blood clotting. This is important to maintain optimal blood flow to the heart, brain, and all other important organs.

Ginkgo and High Blood Pressure

Ginkgo helps to normalize blood pressure by relaxing the artery walls. Natural doctors, such as myself, recommend ginkgo for the treatment of mild to moderate high blood pressure.

Protects the Heart

Ginkgo is effective in protecting heart tissue from the ill effects of free radicals that occur during heart attacks. In a 1995 study that looked at the effects of ginkgo extract injected into oxygen-deprived coronary arteries of rabbits, researchers found that ginkgo significantly reduced the amount of damage to heart tissues.

Improves Blood Flow

Ginkolides B, one of the terpene lactones, inhibits a substance called platelet-activating factor (PAF), thereby improving blood flow.

PAF is a normal part of the healing and clotting process. When one suffers a wound or injury, PAF becomes active in the blood. It stimulates platelets to become sticky and join together to form a clot at the site of the wound. However, too much PAF can lead to sticky blood and restrict blood flow. This can lead to serious diseases such as stroke or peripheral vascular diseases such as intermittent claudication, or reduced circulation to the legs, which can restrict walking.

Platelet–Activating Factor (PAF)
Stimulates the gathering of platelets in the blood to form clots, reducing the flow of blood.

Inhibiting excessive PAF activity, ginkgolide B prevents the abnormal clumping of platelets.

Dosage

Most of the positive studies done with ginkgo have been with a standardized extract that contains 24 percent flavone glycosides and 6 percent terpene lactones. Dosages used in these studies ranged from 120–360 mg daily. I recommend most adults use 180–240 mg daily, taken in divided doses.

Safety

Very few adverse effects have been noted with ginkgo. Less than 1 percent of users report digestive upset. If blood-thinning medications are being taken, ginkgo should be avoided. The use of ginkgo should be discontinued one to two weeks before surgery. Lastly, check with your doctor before combining ginkgo with a class of antidepressants known as MAO inhibitors or blood pressure medicines known as thiazide diuretics.

Cayenne

Cayenne, also known as chili pepper, has been used as a medicinal food for thousands of years. Western herbalists have long used cayenne to treat heart disease and circulatory problems.

Cayenne has mild blood-thinning properties and is a rich source of antioxidant protection against free radicals. It can also reduce cholesterol levels by decreasing intestinal cholesterol absorption and increasing its excretion through the bile as it passes through the digestive tract.

Improves Blood Flow

In studies, cayenne has been shown to decrease abnormal blood clotting by inhibiting the production of thromboxanes. Studies done with people from Thailand who ate chiles on a daily basis found they had increased blood-thinning activity compared with those who consumed a traditional American diet.

Throm-boxanes *Substances that promote blood clotting.*

Artery Cleansing

Laboratory studies have found that cayenne reduces fat deposits in the arteries by enhancing a liver enzyme that metabolizes fat.

Lowers Cholesterol and Triglycerides

Researchers have found that cayenne decreases LDL cholesterol and triglyceride levels. I have not found it to be a potent treatment by itself for elevated cholesterol. However, it can be an important part of a combination herbal formula targeted toward elevated cholesterol and triglyceride levels.

Dosage

For the prevention and treatment of cardiovascular disease, I recommend supplementing a 500-mg capsule or fifteen drops of tincture three times daily.

Safety

Cayenne may cause digestive upset in some people. It should also be used with caution if blood-thinning medication is being taken.

Green Tea

Green tea has a long history of use by the people of China, Japan, and India. It has begun to gain popularity as a beverage in North America, largely because researchers have discovered this tea contains some of the most potent antioxidants known.

Green tea comes from the same leaves of *Camella sinensis* that are used to make black tea. The difference is that green tea undergoes less processing. This reduced processing preserves the antioxidant properties found in green tea. Green tea contains polyphenols, a potent group of antioxidants, whose benefits include prevention of cholesterol oxidation.

A 1992 study found that green tea consumption was a key factor in the longevity of a certain group of Japanese women.

Cardiovascular Disease

A study of 1,371 Japanese men found that high consumption of green tea (ten cups or more) reduced total cholesterol levels while increasing the good HDL cholesterol. The polyphenols in

green tea have been shown to reduce the oxidation of LDL cholesterol.

Dosage

I recommend three or more cups of organic
green tea daily if one has cardiovascular disease.
Of course, this tea can and should be drunk as
part of a comprehensive strategy in preventing
heart disease as well. The active ingredients of
green tea are available in more potent standardized supplement forms so it is not necessary to
drink so much tea. Supplements are available in
tincture or capsule.

Choose organic formulas that contain between
80 and 90 percent polyphenols and 35 and 55
percent epigallocatechin gallate (the strongest of
the polyphenols). Take 250–500 mg of the standardized extract two to three times daily.

Safety

Regular green tea contains approximately 50 mg
of caffeine per cup (while coffee contains 85 mg).
However, offsetting its caffeine content, green tea
also contains an amino acid known as L-theanine,
which has a relaxing effect on the nervous system.
If you are sensitive to caffeine or wish to avoid it,
you can purchase caffeine-free green tea.

Red Yeast Rice Extract

Red yeast rice, the fermented product of rice on
which red yeast (*Monascus purpureus*) has been
grown, is another food supplement with a very
old history of use. Ancient Chinese texts record
the medicinal properties of red yeast rice to improve circulation. It was also used as a food pre-
servative to maintain the color and taste of fish
and meat. Today, it is a dietary staple in China and
Japan and is commonly used by Asians in the
United States.

A powerful supplement, red yeast rice, in well-designed studies, has been shown to significantly lower total cholesterol, LDL cholesterol, and triglyceride levels. In China, the red yeast rice and its effects on cholesterol have been observed in both human and animal studies. It has been shown to reduce cholesterol levels by 11 to 32 percent and triglyceride levels by 12 to 19 percent.

What Makes Red Yeast Rice Effective?

Researchers have found that red yeast rice contains an ingredient called monacolin K, which inhibits the action of an enzyme in the liver (HMG-CoA reductase) that is involved in the synthesis of cholesterol. This is similar to the effects of cholesterol-lowering "statin" drugs such as lovastatin (Mevacor). This similarity has led to some controversy as to whether red yeast rice extract should be considered a dietary supplement or a pharmaceutical. Yet the amount of monacolin K in red yeast rice is quite small (0.2% per 5 mg) compared with the 20–40 mg found in lovastatin. It is thought that other ingredients in red yeast rice may also contribute to its powerful cholesterol-lowering properties. For example, it contains a family of 8 monacolin-related substances that can also inhibit the enzyme HMG-Co A reductase.

Human Studies

In one study, men and women supplemented with 1.2 grams of red yeast extract daily for two months. Researchers found a significant decrease in total and LDL cholesterol. In addition, HDL levels were significantly increased, and elevated triglycerides were found to be lowered.

Also, a double-blind trial at UCLA School of Medicine found that 2.4 grams per day of red yeast rice extract significantly lowered total and LDL cholesterol in a group of people who had

elevated cholesterol after twelve weeks of therapy. In this study, triglycerides were also lowered,
but HDL values did not increase significantly.

Dosage

The amount of red yeast rice extract used in the
studies contained 10–13.5 mg of monacolins per
day. However, FDA regulations do not permit
supplement manufacturers to list the concentration of monacolins in their products. Consumers
will need to contact the manufacturer directly to
learn the concentration of monacolins in order to
take a therapeutic dosage.

Safety

Red yeast may cause some mild side effects such
as heartburn, dizziness, and gas. These symptoms
may only be temporary. Those with a liver disorder should not use red yeast rice extract. Its
safety during pregnancy is unknown, so it should
be avoided. Since red yeast rice extract has a
similar effect on HMG CoA reductase as statin
drugs, it is prudent to take simultaneously 50–100
mg of coenzyme Q_{10}. Studies done on pharmaceutical statin drugs have shown that these medications may contribute to CoQ_{10} deficiencies.

Soy

In the natural health food industry, soy is recog-
nized as a leading food and supplement. It has
been shown to lower total cholesterol and LDL
cholesterol when taken either as a food or supplement. So convincing is the evidence for soy's
beneficial effects on cholesterol that the Food
and Drug Administration approved the claim by
manufacturers that a food containing 6.25 grams
of soy protein had cardiovascular benefits.

Researchers do not yet know the mechanism
for soy's ability to lower cholesterol, but it is

believed that many components of soy, such as the isoflavones, protein, and other constituents are involved.

Lowers Cholesterol and Blood Pressure

An analysis of twenty-nine placebo-controlled studies found that just 31–47 grams of soy protein decreased total cholesterol by 9 percent and LDL cholesterol by 13 percent.

Another study, published in the *American Journal of Clinical Nutrition* in 2002, found that the substitution of soy foods for animal products reduces the risk of coronary artery disease due to reductions in cholesterol, oxidized LDL, homocysteine, and blood pressure.

Prevents LDL Oxidation

One of soy's isoflavones, genistein, was shown in test-tube studies to prevent the oxidation of LDL cholesterol. Researchers also found in one study that the consumption of soy protein over a four-week period led to an eightfold increase in the ability to break down LDL cholesterol.

Dosage

To reduce cholesterol levels, it is recommended that one consume 25 grams or more of soy protein daily. It is important to note that isolated soy isoflavone extract capsules have not been shown to lower cholesterol. Soy foods such as tofu and tempeh, as well as soy protein powder, are effective in reducing cholesterol.

Safety

The most common side effect of soy is digestive upset such as bloating, constipation, or nausea. Soy is one of the more common food sensitivities, so when using it, one should be aware of any changes in digestive function.

CHAPTER 7

NEW RISK MARKERS FOR HEART DISEASE AND THEIR NATURAL SOLUTIONS

In recent years, research into the causes of heart disease has attained greater depth. In the past, cholesterol markers were the primary focus as to the cause of cardiovascular disease. In a nutshell, cholesterol was the villain and the cure was to attack and lower it. Today, we know that elevated cholesterol levels are just one risk factor out of many. Chronic inflammation in the blood vessel walls is now considered to be a more substantial cause of atherosclerosis and the progression of heart disease.

Following, I'll review the newer blood risk markers of heart disease that I discussed in Chapter 1. I recommend that you ask your doctor to order these markers to find out whether you may be at risk, or not. If you find that there is an imbalance with one or more of these markers, you can work with your doctor to decrease your risk. This is best achieved through dietary and lifestyle changes, as well as nutritional supplements. Following is a summary of these markers and corresponding natural protocols that have been proven effective in treating them.

C-Reactive Protein (CRP)

In March 2000, researchers from Harvard University announced that CRP levels were one of the best predictors of future heart attacks and stroke. In fact, a 2002 study published in the

New England Journal of Medicine found that in an analysis of almost 28,000 apparently healthy American women, C-reactive protein level was a stronger predictor of cardiovascular events than the LDL cholesterol level.

CRP is a chemical indicator of the amount of inflammation occurring in the body and blood vessels. Elevated levels of CRP result in a response by the immune system that can lead to the damage of artery walls. Cholesterol and other fatty deposits can lead to hardening and blockage of the arteries.

CRP is known to rise as a result of stealth infections such as chlamydia or Epstein-Barr virus. It is also elevated by the harmful effects of smoking, high blood sugar levels, hypertension, and poor dietary choices.

Natural Solutions

- Eat a diet rich in essential fatty acids, which can be found in flaxseeds, walnuts, and cold-water fish, such as salmon. Plenty of vegetables are also recommended.

- Avoid high glycemic foods such as white bread, muffins, pastries, and other simple sugar products.

- Foods high in saturated fat should be avoided. These include dairy products and fatty red meats.

Supplements

Vitamin E:	400–800 IU daily
Fish oil:	5,000 mg daily
Gamma linoleic acid (GLA):	200–500 mg daily
Bromelain:	500 mg three times daily, between meals

Lipoprotein (a)

Also referred to as Lp(a), this is a more specific cholesterol marker that increases the likelihood of blood clots and plaque formation. This marker is strongly genetic and appears not to be related as much to diet and lifestyle as many of the other risk markers.

Natural Solutions

- Consume a diet low in simple sugars.

- Eat plenty of vegetables and cold-water fish.

Supplements

Niacin (flush free):	3,000 mg daily
Coenzyme Q_{10}:	100–200 mg daily
Policosanol:	20 mg daily
Fish oil:	5,000 mg daily

Homocysteine

The research is very clear. Those with elevated homocysteine levels are at much greater risk for heart disease. Homocysteine is a byproduct of protein metabolism. Due to genetics, some have a tendency to build up this toxic metabolite. B vitamin deficiency is also a common reason that this risk marker becomes dangerously elevated. In addition, low thyroid function can make one more likely to have increased levels of homocysteine.

Natural Solutions

- Reduce the amount of animal protein in the diet and look to vegetable sources such as soy and legumes.

- Increase your intake of fruits and vegetables that are good sources of the B vitamins necessary for homocysteine metabolism.

Supplements

Vitamin B_{12}:   800–2,000 mcg daily

Folic acid: 1–10 mg daily

Vitamin B_6:   20–100 mg daily

Trimethylglycine (TMG):   500–1,000 mg daily

S-Adenosylmethionine
  (SAMe):   400 mg daily

Fibrinogen

Fibrinogen is an important substance involved in blood clotting. However, elevated levels can make one prone to blood clots. It is an independent cardiac risk marker. Fibrinogen tends to be more commonly elevated in smokers, those who are overweight, and those with diabetes.

Natural Solutions

- Avoid simple carbohydrates.

- Consume quality protein sources and plenty of vegetables. Eating cold-water fish has a natural blood-thinning effect and is highly recommended.

Supplements

Fish oil: 5,000–7,000 mg daily

Vitamin E: 400–800 IU daily

Bromelain: 500 mg three times
                            daily, between meals

Garlic: 600 mg daily

Iron

Elevated levels of iron in the body increase the formation of harmful free radicals. This increases the likelihood of an inflammatory response in the blood vessels, as well as cholesterol oxidation.

Consult with your doctor about having your iron levels measured through a blood test.

Natural Solutions

- If your iron levels are elevated, your doctor may recommend a series of blood draws to get the levels down.

Supplements

Avoid taking supplements containing iron if your levels are too high.

Glucose and Insulin

Elevated blood sugar (glucose) levels and corresponding insulin levels increase free-radical formation and blood vessel inflammation. This is not seen only in people with diabetes. People who have a condition known as insulin resistance experience a spiking of glucose and insulin levels, which means that cells are not accepting the insulin (which transports the glucose) efficiently.

Natural Solutions

- Those with high glucose levels should be on an insulin resistant diet, also known as the "Syndrome X" diet, which is low in high glycemic foods. It should include quality protein sources such as fish, legumes, soy, and lean poultry, as well as plenty of vegetables.

Supplements

Chromium:	400–1,000 mcg daily
Vanadium:	100 mg daily
B complex:	100 mg daily
Magnesium:	500 mg daily
Gymnemma sylvestre (25 percent):	600 mg daily

High Blood Pressure

Aside from the various blood markers discussed here, high blood pressure is one of the biggest contributors to heart disease. The increased pressure inside the artery walls causes inflammation and damage. If the problem goes untreated for long periods of time, it also can lead to damage of the heart muscle.

Natural Solutions

- Consume a diet that is rich in minerals such as potassium, magnesium, and calcium—these can be found in fresh fruits and vegetables and their juices.

- People who are overweight are more susceptible to high blood pressure. These people may have insulin resistance and should follow a diet that reduces simple carbohydrates.

- Water intake is important as low levels of dehydration can contribute to elevated blood pressure.

- Regular exercise and stress-reduction techniques can be quite important in the natural treatment of this disease. Both should be done on a daily basis.

Supplements

Coenzyme Q_{10}:	100–200 mg daily
Magnesium:	500 mg daily
Calcium:	1,000 mg daily
Hawthorn:	900 mg daily
Potassium:	200–300 mg daily

Chronic Infections

Chronic, low-grade infections in the body are being linked as a possible risk factor for the development of heart disease. Small bacteria and yeast overgrowth may cause inflammation in blood vessels, setting up an inflammatory response. Research is preliminary but continued studies may show a significant connection.

A healthy range is still being determined by researchers.

Natural Solutions

Oregano oil:	500 mg three times daily
Echinacea:	500 mg three times daily
Garlic:	600–900 mg daily

CONCLUSION

Today, heart disease remains the number-one killer of all Americans. With an aging population, one can expect the number of people to develop cardiovascular disease to skyrocket. However, the reality is that heart disease can be prevented and treated with dietary and lifestyle changes, and with the therapeutic aid of targeted nutritional supplements.

As it turns out, elevated cholesterol levels are only a part of the picture when it comes to cardiovascular risk markers. The most up-to-date scientific research shows that chronic inflammation in the blood vessels is the most serious threat to cardiovascular health. A blood marker of inflammation known as C-reactive protein is the best measurable predictor of heart disease risk. In addition, newer blood markers, many of which are genetic in origin, are great predictors of heart disease risk. Homocysteine, lipoprotein (a), fibrinogen, and others have turned out to be more important independent risk markers than cholesterol. Levels of these newer markers need to be tested if you are to become proactive in re - ducing or stopping the devastating effects these factors can have on the cardiovascular system. Once you know where your cardiovascular weaknesses lie, nutritional and supplemental means can help you to avoid or lessen their effects.

I have discussed how diet affects the health of

one's heart and circulatory system. The reduction of simple sugars and harmful fats combined with an increased intake of vegetables, healthy fats, and quality proteins can have a profound effect on your cardiovascular health.

Several nutritional supplements have been proven to be of tremendous value in preventing and treating heart disease. Herbs such as guggul and red yeast rice extract are also very effective. In addition, antioxidants such as vitamins E and C, coenzyme Q_{10}, and several others discussed in this book are invaluable in preventing damage to the heart and arteries.

Policosanol is a breakthrough supplement that safely and effectively reduces cholesterol and other genetic markers of heart disease. It has a remarkably protective effect on the cardiovascular system without potential toxic effects found with many cholesterol-lowering pharmaceuticals. And its cholesterol-lowering effects compare favorably with these same drugs. In addition, Policosanol does not deplete coenzyme Q_{10} levels, a concern with "statin" cholesterol drugs.

Policosanol has also been shown effective in the treatment of angina and intermittent claudication. This is also a valuable supplement for the prevention of stroke. Since Policosanol is one of the most well-studied natural products in the world, one can feel confident in its efficacy and its safety.

Exercise and stress reduction are other essentials in any program designed to prevent and treat heart disease. Plan to make them a part of your regular activity schedule.

In all, it is important that we educate ourselves regarding the benefits of a holistic approach to a healthy heart. Nature has provided us with all the medicines we need to stay healthy. By availing ourselves of these responsibly, we can live life to the fullest.

SELECTED
REFERENCES

Arruzazabala ML, Molina V, Mas R, Fernandez L, Carbajal D, Valdes S, Castano G. Antiplatelet effects of policosanol (20 and 40 mg/day) in healthy volunteers and dyslipidaemic patients. Clin Exp Pharmacol Physiol 2002 Oct;29(10): 891–7.

Arruzazabala ML, Noa M, Menendez R, Mas R, Carbajal D, Valdes S, Molina V. Protective effect of policosanol on atherosclerotic lesions in rabbits with exogenous hypercholesterolemia. Braz J Med Biol Res 2000 Jul;33(7): 835–40.

Arruzazabala ML, et al. Comparative study of policosanol, aspirin and the combination therapy policosanol-aspirin on platelet aggregation in healthy volunteers. Pharmacol Res 1997;36:293–7.

Batiste MC, Schaefer EJ. Diagnosis and management of lipoprotein abnormalities. Nutr Clin Care 2002 May-Jun;5(3):115–23.

Castano G, Mas R, Fernandez L, Fernandez JC, Illnait J, Lopez LE, Alvarez E. Effects of polico - sanol on postmenopausal women with type II hypercholesterolemia. Gynecol Endocrinol 2000 Jun;14(3): 187–95.

Castano G, Mas R, Arruzazabala ML, Noa M, Illnait J, Fernandez JC, Molina V, Menendez A. Effects of policosanol and pravastatin on lipid profile, platelet aggregation and endothelemia in older hypercholesterolemic patients. *Int J Clin Pharmacol Res* 1999;19(4):105–16.

Fernandez L et al. "Policosanol:Results of a post-marketing surveillance study of 27,879 patients." *Curr. Ther. Res.* 1998; 59:7717–22.

Gouni-Berthold I, Berthold HK. Policosanol: clinical pharmacology and therapeutic significance of a new lipid-lowering agent. *Am Heart J* 2002 Feb;143(2):356–65.

Heber D, Yip I, Ashley JM, et al. Cholesterol-lowering effects of a proprietary Chinese red-yeast-rice dietary supplement. *Am J Clin Nutr* 1999; 69:231–6.

Jenkins DJ, Kendall CW, Jackson CJ, Connelly PW, Parker T, Faulkner D, Vidgen E, Cunnane SC, Leiter LA, Josse RG. Effects of high- and low-isoflavone soyfoods on blood lipids, oxidized LDL, homocysteine, and blood pressure in hyperlipidemic men and women. *Am J Clin Nutr* 2002 Aug;76(2):365–72.

Kishi T, Kishi H, and Folkers K. Inhibition of cardiac CoQ_{10} enzymes by clinically used drugs and possible prevention. In: Biomedical and Clinical Aspects of Coenzyme Q, Vol. I. Folkers K and Yamamura (eds). Elsevier/North Holland Biomedical Press, Amsterdam, 1977; pp. 47–62.

Kurl S, Tuomainen TP, Laukkanen JA, Nyyssonen K, Lakka T, Sivenius J, Salonen JT. Plasma vitamin C modifies the association between hypertension and risk of stroke. *Stroke.* 2002 Jun;33(6): 1568–73.

Niyanand S et al. Clinical trials with guggulipid: A new hypolipidemic agent. *Journal of the Association of Physicians of India* 1989;37(5): 323–328.

Plotnick GD, Corretti MC, Vogel RA. Effect of antioxidant vitamins on the transient impairment of endothelium-dependent brachial artery vaso-activity following a single high-fat meal. *JAMA* 1997 Nov 26;278(20):1682–6.

Prat H, et al. Comparative effects of policosanol and two HMG-CoA reductase inhibitors on type II hypercholesterolemia. Published in Spanish. *Rev Med Chile* 1999;127:286–94.

Ridker PM, Rifai N, Rose L, Buring JE, Cook NR. Comparison of C-reactive protein and low-density lipoprotein cholesterol levels in the prediction of first cardiovascular events. *N Engl J Med* 2002 Nov 14;347(20):1557–65.

Tauchert M et al. Effectiveness of hawthorn extract LI 132 compared with captopril. *Munch Medizinische Wochenschrift* 1994;136:27–33.

Wang J, Lu Z, Chi J, et al. Multicenter clinical trial of the serum lipid-lowering effects of a *Monascus purpureus* (red yeast) rice preparation from traditional Chinese medicine. *Curr Ther Res* 1997;58: 964–77.

Weikl A et al. Crataegus special extracts WS 1442. Objective proof of effectiveness for patients with heart failure (NYHA II). *Fortschritte Medizin* 1996;114(24):291–296.

OTHER BOOKS
AND RESOURCES

Stengler, Mark. *The Natural Physician's Healing Therapies.* Paramus, NJ: Prentice Hall Press, 2001.

Stengler, Angela and Mark. *Your Menotype, Your Menopause.* Paramus, NJ: Prentice Hall Press, 2002.

Challem, Jack. *Syndrome X: The Complete Nutritional Program to Prevent and Reverse Insulin Resistance.* John Wiley and Sons, 2001.

GreatLife Magazine
Consumer magazine with articles on vitamins, minerals, herbs, and foods.
Available for free at many health and natural food stores.

Let's Live Magazine
Consumer magazine with emphasis on the health benefits of vitamins, minerals, and herbs.
Customer service:
1-800-676-4333
P.O. Box 74908
Los Angeles, CA 90004
Subscriptions: 12 issues per year, $19.95 in the U.S.; $31.95 outside the U.S.

Physical Magazine

Magazine oriented to body builders and other serious athletes.

Customer service:
1-800-676-4333
P.O. Box 74908
Los Angeles, CA 90004

Subscriptions: 12 issues per year, $19.95 in the U.S.; $31.95 outside the U.S.

The Nutrition Reporter™ newsletter

Monthly newsletter that summarizes recent medical research on vitamins, minerals, and herbs.

Customer service:
P.O. Box 30246
Tucson, AZ 85751-0246
e-mail: jack@thenutritionreporter.com
www.nutritionreporter.com

Subscriptions: $26 per year (12 issues) in the U.S.; $32 U.S. or $48 CNC for Canada; $38 for other countries.

Websites

Medline

http://www.ncbi.nlm.nih.gov/entrez/query
For specific medical journal abstracts.

National Center for Complementary and Alternative Medicine, National Institutes of Health (NIH)

http://nccam.nih.gov/nccam
Search a database of 180,000 bibliographic citations regarding complementary and alternative therapies extracted from MEDLINE.

Office of Dietary Supplements, National Institutes of Health

http://dietary-supplements.info.nih.gov

Scientific resources (including recent research findings regarding supplements), general information about supplements, and programs and activities of the Office of Dietary Supplements.

INDEX

9 781681 628660